The Blue Cardigan

~By~

S Thuam Siam Ngaihte

ISBN: 9798547187261

The Blue Cardigan

Acknowledgment

I wanted to thank my wife *Ching Ngaihte*, my children *Mung Ngaihte* and *Kim Ngaihte* for their support and understanding of my time at the computer.

Table of Contents

Prologue

Her social media post reflected her mind. He must have been reading it. He wants to fly like a bird in the sky – free from all the toxics of life. His heavy heart always weighed him down. I suggested he could simply go back. He told me it ain't as easy as it appears. We have our own life, journey, and the people we met.

The scene at home was different now. He felt lost. No one needs him. But there's also a possibility that he did not pour out his heart enough.

He's been through a lot. If his time in the Golden Triangle could not change him. I don't think I could. He's a roamer.

But then he reiterated his love for his wife did not change – she gained more freedom. Then again I told him she might not enjoy her freedom.

'Yes, maybe or maybe not!'

He did not want to go deep right now.

But soon he will. He has to. No, he's unpredictable. I cannot say anything about his future. He is kicking his ball. Not me.

'Fine by me!' I said to him. The deafening sound of the traffic seems to agree with me. This time it becomes louder. Many are rushing home. They have their home and are eager to get home.

He is not one of them. I'm afraid it might be now or never. Yet it's better if someone not to draw a quick conclusion on anything. Nothing is over until our very last breathe. Many times it is more of our attitude which matters the most.

~1~

Lunchtime

The hot, wet, and humid monsoon season has just passed. The weather is pleasant mostly in the morning. It also stays cool with a breeze of air flowing through the streets. The streets had once witnessed the dry and desert-like heatwaves a few months ago.

Now we're nearing the smell of extreme cold once again. Just outside our workplace were some of the trees whose leaves are yellowing as they prepare for winter. The view and the weather are pleasant except for the deafening sounds of traffic who were trying to find a way on the roads.

It is during this time when during our lunch hour, we'd escape from the concrete structure to get a glimpse of all those similar yet scenic happenings on the front side of our office. I am new to this workplace although I have worked for some time in another workplace, some of which are not related to my present job.

As I am new to this place, I acted slowly in making friends. It's a different scenario than my previous workplace. I met different kinds of people here – both younger and older or senior workers.

While some of them were quick in passing judgment about our different traditions and culture including our choice of food during our lunchtime. But we have one thing in common. We need rest, a quiet time to escape from our daily routine of working hard. This short lunchtime is meant to be escapist.

'You looked different today,' I said to my colleague who was already there standing in the driveway under the shade of that small tree. Not everyone came for this spot every day.

Looking beyond him, I saw the gas station on the other side of the road getting their customers in good numbers. It must a good day for them, I simply said in my mind.

"What do you mean by that?" he replied profusely after some time. His weird smile turning into laughter. I don't know what will come next nor do I want to draw his attention that much. I thought it to be a conversation starter and I meant it that way.

'You must be talking about my *blue cardigan.....*' his tone did not change.

I don't know whether it is a question thrown back at me or simply accepting my compliment. So, I simply nodded.

Suddenly he burst out laughing which followed him singing few lines of his favorite song from a Bollywood movie. I don't know what to say next. I waited.

His eyes appeared deep to me. There must be stories inside him which is not made known to me. But as a man, I'm not afraid of whatever happens next. He kept on singing after every puff of his cigarette. I don't like the smell of cigarettes, it makes me nauseous. So, I try to move away from him. He knew it.

'Stay, simply sit here. Lunchtime is not over yet.' He told me. I move a bit further yet I did not hesitate. It is my first interaction with him. He is very much a senior to me in this workplace particularly.

'Why is everyone complimenting when I wear this blue cardigan?' he continued. This time I did not answer. I have the intuition now that he will answer himself in a moment. So I endure the awkward silence while checking messages and engaging myself in some other things.

'My wife gifted this to me, " he said. "It's a long time back now.'

'She must have a good taste of shirts and sweaters for you.'

Except for his vague smile which he often did there seems to be a good charisma inside him. He talks a bit about life which I realized I will hear more often from him if we continue to meet during lunchtime. We did not talk about personal or family matters inside the workplace. There are several reasons for that. These were very private matters to us. We don't want our family matters exposed or intrude into the atmosphere of the workplace.

Next, we want to maintain distance from everyone. I don't know if other genders of our colleagues also feel the same. Yet I expected they would as I did the same. There is a different workplace personality and behavior at home.

No workplace stress needs to be brought home not its influence on our behavior should be appreciated. It's a different world and living in this short span of life. The workplace atmosphere must be left behind as we enter our home.

'Yes, she did,' said he affirmatively.

We talked about few things but not about his wife nor my family and upbringing. Instead, we talked about the happenings around us. I discovered that he is not that much into politics. Most of our conversation hit a dead end immediately one after another. So. We keep on jumping topics over and over. I did enjoy this kind of conversation. Yet I stayed.

I wanted to go back and asked about his wife and all the story behind his **blue cardigan**. But then he hesitated. He simply dismissed it as one among the daily needs they bought as a husband and a wife. So, I try to maintain the limited wiring around it.

But then my instinct coerced me to at least asked a thing about his reaction while his blue cardigan became the focal point. And as we were listening to his old jokes I tried to poke him with a question which he might not be willing to hear.

'Your cardigan looks fresh, did you only get it, as a gift, only last year? I asked.

This time Jag gave me a weird look. His name is long so we simply called him Jag. Most of the time, we did not address our colleagues in our full name or as written in our Identity Card to ease out friction in making wrongful pronunciation and saving time. While some prefer to be addressed that way only because they do not want to reveal their real name in front of everyone with whom they did not get acquainted.

I can sense his unwillingness to give me a one-line reply. He hardly did that. Most of his answers never came. So I try to cover it up with a joke which he didn't take it well either.

It's not easy, baggage to carry on
Love is baggage to carry on
Love carries me on to move on
If our glass heart could crack.... is one of his
songs.

He looked at his wristwatch and signaled us to resume our work as our lunchtime is over for a day.

After that day we did not talk about personal things. It was a mistake on his part to almost let it off on that day. Well, that's how I took it. Another thing might be that he is willing to tell his stories. I saw a little frustration inside him besides work pressure. Should we talk about work pressure then we would surely hit it off, gossiping about others although it would hardly serve us any good. Further, if somebody overheard our conversation it would result in putting us together on a different sphere inside our workplace.

Yet he tried to bring back his issues which I ignored most of the time. I saw something different in him. His penchant for old Bollywood songs with meaningful lyrics says something about him. There is an emptiness inside him. He is hiding it all this time. I don't know how long he's been doing it.

Some days he is very positive but the other day he is not. In my new workplace, I did not want to mingle with people whom I did not know well.

So, to put it short, I'm also just passing my time by not taking someone seriously yet I would like to build a friendship if there's someone who could also bail me out if I face difficulties in the workplace.
But for now, I did not see him as that kind of person. He seems lonely in the crowded world. I love stories and exploring people if they are willing. I saw him as someone who is willing to tell his stories but does not know how to.

~**2**~

Self Conscious

I started making friends in the workplace by now. Some of them advise not to hang out with him. He is alone most of the time, they'd told me. That I can also see from the very beginning.

The other day he wore his blue cardigan again. It doesn't make any difference for most of us. All of our colleagues, although they had different sets of shirts and trousers, *kurti* or *kurtas*, we wear our favorites most of the time. Some are even recognized by the color and stripes of their shirt.

But for Jag, every time he wore his blue cardigan he seems to be self-conscious. It might be because of my compliment once in a while and the story behind it. I too become curious about it. He has never mentioned his wife except for that day. And I don't want to ask about it either because I'm afraid it makes him uncomfortable. Maybe his wife passed away, left him, divorced him, or was not in contact with him.

The thing is I don't want to hurt somebody's sentiments without me being careless about what I speak. Nor do I wanted to invade the privacy of others just as I do not want others to do it to me. I let out a little – the iceberg of almost everything. Oh, by the way, you can call me Sam. Sorry for the late introduction. This might not be my real name but does it matter? I don't think so.

When one of my colleagues Tanu saw us talking few times in a week, she advised me not to interact much with my newfound friend. No, I cannot call him my friend. Not yet! It was only for 10-15 minutes during our lunchtime.

Once in a while, we would visit the eatery joints nearby our workplace with the younger generations of our workplace. Women in particular are very much aware of people around them. They only talk to people with whom they feel safe and especially with co-workers, if in a workplace, who would not pass on the gossips and information they'd probably share.

Tanu is witty, self-compose, and carries herself very well in the workplace. I also believe she would do well in her family and society. She is strictly professional and not hesitant onto passing what she thought is good. She simply did not talk to everybody nor does she talk to me very often. She knows how to maintain distance. If I may add more - she is well balanced in her perception of life.

Well, this is all about and a short introduction of Tanu. She lends her voice when she feels necessary so I think I owe her an introduction in the least. Since I'm new to the workplace at that time, she is a bit protective over me. That is why she advised me to keep out from Jag as she sees him as he might influence me to things I did know experienced. I think she already knows something about the person we're talking to. Yet I'm willing to explore more as if I can do something in return. But I wasn't sure either.

'We got married,' he told me. 'We were in love, enjoyed our honeymoon somewhere in the hill stations,' he continued. This time I'm not that interested. So I tried to cut him off several times.

'I'm also married. We did the same thing,' I replied. ' It's nothing new for a man to do it.' When someone reached a marriageable age we're on the lookout. Although we don't intend to tie the knot with whoever crosses our way. We try our best to find the right person. A person of integrity would reserve himself or herself for their future partner. It is nothing noble but the right thing to do as a person.

Jag wanted to say something more but could find time on that day. His trademark vague smile once again wrinkled up his face but disappear quickly as if nothing had happened. We went back to our workplace for another half of the day.

'Yes, I'm coming! I'm outta my way. I shouted as try to walk out of the house,' he said. He pretended to be someone calling him whenever he wanted to. He told me he wanted to spend more time outside the house with his gang of friends. Some of the things before he got married are still at large. He wasn't ready for a lifestyle change.

'Did you not talk about it before?' I quipped. 'We did….,' he said with a long pause. There is a deep thought today.

I waited.

'That's how I first started,' he continued at last with a huge sigh of relief. But I can see the pain in his eyes. What did you start for, I wanted to ask but I believe he will reveal it in due course. For now, he just needed someone who'd simply nodded his head and listen to his story.

No one called him but there is frustration inside him. His dear wife is now busy with their child. There is no time left for him. She thought that he would understand her. But he still had his longing unsatisfied due to the change in the situation. She thought her husband must be happy since she bore him a child. And this might be the new addition to their small family.

Their perception of life becomes different day by day. Her wife thought she was losing time to focus on her career once again. Their love sometimes doesn't felt enough. They need to think about their future. He brought home money enough for them to live on.

I kept half-listening to his story today. So I can recollect a few of them – only this much. One more thing, I don't see a point in listening to this not-so-encouraging story. I want some other jokes to refresh my mind during this short period of rejuvenation. But somehow I am drawn to his story so far. I hope it turns out to be good in the end. Yet I am still unsure if I could listen to him anymore.

'There is an atmosphere of frustration in the home,' he said in a low voice to me the next week. He appeared to be sober. 'Uh-huh, go on your way to redemption!' I said to him today. I don't know if I sound harsh to him. I might. But I don't want to bother.

'One day I will be recollecting your narration. And I might turn into a small book if you keep telling me your story.' Then I pause. He took out his cigarette which he knew I don't like. We remain silent for a while.

Just then Tanu appeared in the scene. She has some work in the nearby office for which she was going alone. So, I offered to accompany her. Jag knew the situation.

'Sam, I'll treat you a cup of juice tomorrow,' he said all of a sudden.

'Fine!'

So I went with Tanu for a change that day. We had a hearty laugh as we shared what goes wrong in our workplace where we are directly or indirectly involved. We came to some of them are done with a purpose. But not beyond the solutions, we can provide nor will it harm the workplace we represented.

She continued to warn me about Jag because our senior have rumors going on about him in the past. Someone claimed to have heard of his failed marriage and his failed relationship even after that.

Jag is not someone who appeared to have so many stories behind him if you met him for the very first time.

'So what do you discussed with him? I often see you standing with him,' she asked.

'Nothing much. We guys like to talk about everything. From politics to sports, to cooking, and the likes,' I replied.

She tried to believe me. Yet she laughed at me with disbelief.

' You are a good person, you have other friends to talk to. So, spend less time with him,' she continued. I agree with her. But the loneliness in his eyes stuck in my mind. I might not be able to help him.

More than that I was afraid that I might make things worse for him. If any untoward incident occurs I might be the one to blame. He is putting up in a small paid lodging in the city where he is a veteran now, they told me.

Since it can paint a bad picture or personality on me by interacting with women co-workers, I chose to avoid them as well. For a married person, there were simple yet important things to take care of.

A little gossip about my behavior at the workplace may reach home soon. Every little act of me is to salvage a projected life-long and healthy relationship with the one I love.

Further, I did not entertain calls of any type from my co-workers when I'm at home. It is better to leave the work-related matter at the workplace. I did not want anyone to affect my time at home with my children. I don't want to apologize for being unprepared during any call while I'm at home. I have the right to remain in peace at least in my small world.

Jag listened to me while I narrated all these things. He looked bored. But I did not care about him. In my mind, I was saying you too speak of yourself the way you like.

'Thank you for listening to me,' he hurled at me as if I'm doing something wrong. He tried leaving the spot hurriedly. But he came back.

He recalled his frustration at home many years ago. 'Are you still frustrated?' I asked.

'Oh, you knew very little about me. But if I don't leave this job you'll get to know more, he continued. I hate it when somebody told me that I knew very little about them.

Is it an excuse or their way of saying does it bother you? It's my life. Well, no one can know the other person too much about them even though we might seem to be very close.

'Fine by me!' I replied.

Since you came back why not talked about your previous frustration before our lunchtime is over. He looked at his wristwatch and gave me a blank reply. Then slowly he started talking again. I signaled him to go on.

Jag told me that his wife was too busy for him. He appreciates her taking care of the house while he was away searching for food. But his occasional outing with his friends makes his wife frustrate him. She hardly talked to him when he gets home.

He knew she wasn't happy with how things are going. But he did not like her reaction. He wanted to keep things low but sometimes lost control of himself. So, he'd rushed out of their home in the middle of their argument.

Every argument matters in marriage. But leaving in the middle of it makes things worse. That is because without the matter being settled they hardly visit again. And the worst part is it will surely surface out once again.

'How can you leave home just like that? I interrupted.

'It's just occasional. I stay put because I love my wife. I did not run out. Not yet!'

Now I have a feeling that this man was leaving home somewhere in his past. But I'm not sure how long or did he really did it. I don't want to confront him.

He doesn't appear to be that kind of a person. Inside our workplace, he is sincere and hardworking. He did his best. And sometimes very towards everyone. So I dare not assume he left home to live alone in the city.

'She did well enough,' he continued. 'But our frustration hugely affected our marriage and the atmosphere of the house. I don't want that kind of atmosphere for my child to grow up.'

I did not ask him the name of his wife till this time. And I don't intent to know more about it either. But it seems that they have a simple yet difficult phase in their family.

He goes on mumbling something indistinctly. He takes out his cigarette while he glanced at me as if he is saying sorry. Then he lit it up and carefully released the smoke so that it does not wane towards me.

'I could have reacted well. But my heart did the opposite. My wife gives less interest in me.

I don't know whether it's because her attitude towards me gets changed nor do I know she had less knowledge or interest to face the cloud of frustration looming large inside our home.'

'Maybe she thought you'd better understand the situation and what to do next,' I added.

He nodded. But did not appear to agree with me either. He signaled our co-workers must be wondering about us. He begged me not to let anyone knew about the conversation we just had.

~3~

Frustration

I'm not sure about the probable outcome of our small talks. But I decided to hear him out as far he wanted to talk. This must be holding too much inside him. I simply said to me if he lets it out he might get a sigh of relief from his current state of mind. At the same time, I do not show any interest in his story.

The other day, we met again in the same place, under the shade. The Corporation who looked after the area installed some cemented stool in the front patio of our Office building. As per my calculations, I don't think the many workers around our area would sit on those concrete stools or elevated areas in the hot summer wind.

However, now that winter is approaching I think people will flock to this area to sit under the sun. But this around it has very few takers except for the few roamers in the city who would take rest for a while here.

Among them you can see different kinds of people who spend their time, hardly talking to each other.

This time again, Jag continued his story I acted as if I don't want more of it. But he was adamant to listen. So he continued resuming about the frustration inside his home and marriage. I tried to interrupt him several times by asking him whether they go to a counselor or not. He never bothers to give me a reply.

By now, he simply focussed on working hard, he told me. He put good food on the table without expecting too much from his wife. However, the flash of romantic vibes is decreasing day by day. We hardly talk to each other although we laughed it was like never before or at least to me.

'My wife seems to like the new development,' he told me looking at the sky. I'm not sure what he meant by that. By now his job is simply to put food on the table.

He went home late in the night mostly during those periods. But since they are not talking much, there is less friction in their relationship. For someone who did not see the internal things, everything would appear normal to them.

There is less nagging in the house. But then he realized they're taking a wrong stand on their commitment. They are simply waiting for the other to falter so that the other would blame him or her for everything that is going wrong before.

It doesn't last long. We simply can't wait. We're two peoples who are in love before. I wanted to give her respect. Yet going by the way how we try to find peace in the house, which he doubts it. They don't recognize their love languages anymore.

'It must be a happy marriage, eh!' I quipped. His blank look gave me a lot of answers. There is a huge void in their marriage. I want to know what he did next. But I waited for him to reveal it in his time. I don't want to rush him.

By now I have this assumption that if I could go on revisiting the past life that hurts him so much he might get some sort of healing. I read from a book healing life hurts. You have to revisit all the scars which you think you've forgotten to face one by one without simply allowing them to resurface since you do not uproot them. They are still stuck to your life but deep enough to be hidden. You live in fear that it might explode somewhere at any given time.

He went home late. He acted like a child. No, it's both of them. He spent most of his time away from home. When he does not have reasons to go out, he'd simply created a scene or acted as if someone is calling him. He now prefers boardgame with his friends over time with his family.

Before he knows he is running away slowly from his home. In its entirety, he doesn't blame himself. He gives less importance to the upkeeping of their child. Pity eyes he can see in their child. This is not how he wanted things to take shape.

Then he looked at his wife. She is unhappy but she doesn't create a scene. It's a shame for the neighbors to hear them shouting at each other. The situation now is not good but nothing of the shouts and scene happens. Their neighbors might be thinking they are rebuilding their lives.

However, deep inside there is something hidden that might explode sooner or later. They did not spend time together. And the worst part is they don't seem to bother that much. Time will heal everything they believed in but time is ticking fast. No changes can be seen.

They are simply not talking to each other.

While I did not concur with everything, I have heard certain people that in the second or third year of marriage, there's some kind of frustration in the relationship. It's just that relationship is taking its root deeper. I told him that they could overcome if they work together. Every day is not a smooth ride. There's a bright future waiting for them.

I try to cheer him up by reminding one of the newspaper articles we read the other day. In the paper, it shocked the people who attend the marriage ceremony of a certain couple because the groom simply runaway placing his attire on her bride. While there's a movie made of The Runaway Bride, it's rare to see the groom running away from the spot.

In my younger years, I heard about a lady who simply said 'NO' instead of the highly anticipated 'I do' in the ceremony arrange for them. Since it's a rare case, I saw her as very daring. However, should I have access to her real state of mind, I might pity her. It's a bizarre situation nevertheless.

Now, Jag was smiling at him sheepishly looking at himself.

'Are you wishing you did that too?' I smiled at him too.

'You bet...,' he said bursting out into one of his empty laughter.

After a while, he continued narrating the situation in his little home. By now poor Jag made the mistake of assuming that his wife is happy just the way they're living. Truly speaking, they're not. It's just that there's no one to break the ice. Love can no longer wax cold at night. Yet they acted their part. They lacked passion or intimate relationships. Worst, no one is eager to admit it. They stand on the wrong foot.

When he is telling all about this past development in their house I don't want to listen anymore. Yet he persisted.

'Wow wow wow!' Mister, I'm hearing only one side of the story. You cannot backstab on someone you love dearly,' I said at last.

As usual, he gives me no quick reply. He hummed away with one of his melodious songs turning away from me. His songs are meaningful. This is the only thing I like about him.

Talking about songs - I love listening to meaningful songs. I love intriguing lyrics. I love words. I wanted to delve into the world of the writer or composer when I came across beautiful songs. For me, music is the added spice of words enhancing the taste. More than that I am more into the wordings, the scene, and what the lyricist would like to portray. Many of us miss the element the writer wants to portray.

At times, Jag was accused of having relationships outside his marriage. That I cannot tell you in its entirety. But looking at how they stand at home. It is one among those encounters of a person who runs away from his responsibilities. He hardly spends time at home.

Yet he assured me that he never drink from another well. He only drinks from his well. Many times he finds it difficult to drink from his well. It doesn't sweet like before was one among his comments. I don't want to go deep on that. So I simply believed him. I also assured him that I believed him in this matter. He doesn't need to talk more about it.

However, it becomes a matter of concern to his wife more and more. Maybe it was because she wants to draw attention to raise her voice. Women should be able to raise their voices. No, not shouting. They should be given space to speak their mind. Yet as you see the situation here, the time is never ripe for their full conversation. Time is ticking. No one wants to be the one who set off the bomb. They were unable to express their love.

Over and over he started hearing complaints when he reached home. The lay-off phase of their plane is almost over. Soon they will be back to their original self. Both of them are not willing to board it. But no one is ready to change their stand. They were afraid their plane might catch fire mid-air. Fear is in their mind. Still, they don't change for good.

Jag told me that he often started staying out from home. He cannot recall how exactly did he spend those days. It takes a toll on him. Sometimes, he sleeps outside the house although he went home.

He doesn't feel like going to bed. Their bed of roses had turned into a bed of thorns! How can I sleep among the thorns? He admitted that the same way must be for his wife.

They lived in poverty – the poverty of love and affection. There is a glass door between them. It might break anytime soon. Distance becomes the issue of their living.

~4~

Dragging Along

He admitted that he was dragging along just like for too long. His helplessness leads him to think that silence is the better way to deal with the current situation at home. It's mostly because he was not interested in almost everything when his business suffered a setback.

One of his acquaintances in the land dealing business was plotting another project which would exclude him. His long dream of setting up a local enterprise where a complex would be set up for anyone to open their shop seems to go down the drain.

I can see from his eyes that he was very committed and interested in the said project. When he looked at the vast empty land he saw the developing neighborhood in the area. Due to the recent infighting between some ethnicity in the surrounding area, many residents lost their homes. They were simply residing in a rented home in the corner of the town.

Before the influx of the tourist, he wanted to give them a facelift. They are privileged to live in a place where tourists wanted to visit them. It implies their hometown must have a good environment and beautiful landscape. If someone bothers to visit the corner part of the town it would be a shame for the community as a whole.

Yet his plan was not only for upliftment, it was also for business purposes. It was a two-way plan which would benefit him and the town dwellers especially those living in rented places.

He goes on to tell me that his problem in the workplace did not interest his woman. He felt threatened – someday he might not be able to put food on the table.

Anita was not interested in this ongoing problem faced by his man on the work front. Maybe she was not interested or she does not have the knowledge to go over with him. He brought home the laid-out plan. Still, she was adamant to at least listen to it.

He needs someone who listens to him. Not giving him solutions but just someone to talk to. Not only that she warned him not to lose money. They have to help her brothers who are stuck in some kind of debt. Every season at home did not go well at this time.

So he continued to seek some other things from outside the house. I did not agree with him when he told me this. But as he told me many times, I was just trying to be that person who is listening to him.

'There must be something you too must have missed about your woman,' I quipped at last.

The look on his face is not the one you would like to see from a man. I do not want him to be angry or feel bad about me. Anyway, he is of great help to me in the workplace. He is a rescuer – his seniority I can use the most. I have learned lots of things about handling workplace politics from him.

All of us had a good side attached to us. It's not that onetime meeting, experience, or saying you heard about someone all the time. There can be a contrasting personality to every person. This I learn from my meeting with Jag.

Then he told me that while they were dating his woman, she is always cheerful – 'this beautiful lady would light up my world forever' – was his thought which captivated his heart. Till today, she did not lose being cheerful. But they now know each other deeper than before.

Gifting each other gifts somehow lighten up the atmosphere in their house. His concern during that period was whether they were going too much on material things. Our emotion tanky ado does not fully get filled by material things, it wants something more than that. Yet we also have to admit that material things do make us happy at some level. However, too much materialism is a threat in different aspects of life.

Simply treating husbands as bosses or husbands only trying to rule over their women is a weakness in both ways. Everything should stem out of love and respect and not out of fear in a relationship.

She is the woman of his dream. He fondly talks of the time they spent together. Those good days are lost – they might not be regained any time soon. That's his hope.

But just dragging along without addressing the mounting gap between them would cause irreparable damage soon.

Till now they were unable to recreate the magic of their romance, which is dying soon. They are staring into the darkness of time – they need something to light them up – a spark of their romance needs to be reignited.

ॐॐॐ

~**5**~

Trouble in Paradise

One night as he stood there thinking whether to enter the house or stay out of it again, he decided not to disturb the peace of the home where his beloved wife and children are sleeping. He saw himself as the cause of trouble in their small paradise.

He thought he did the right thing when he turns back towards the dark again. He soon disappeared into the dark of the night. 'Part of me has died there on that night.....,' he said.

I give him time to recollect himself back in the present. I'm saddened to hear his story. But I want to know more about what happens next. I don't want him to tell me. It made me wonder how this good soul ended up just like that.

That night as he headed back to the town... He stopped right there, not willing to share more. I can feel with him. And, as I offered to console him, he was adamant about it. It revealed he was still hurt from what had happened before. He needs time.

He told me he lost all the stages of love. One, newfound love in his wife keeps him happy. Yet he was unable to hold onto it. Second, He settled too quickly - both in their minds and character. Third, they were unable to keep the spark of their love keeps glowing. Fourth, both were busy with their work or in their venture of life. Fifth, the ship was left to sail by itself – not giving enough care in their emotions. Sixth, their past life get back to them – I don't ask more about this issue.

'Enough!' I said. 'You could seek help at that time.'

He admitted he did wrong but he told me he was simply helpless at the time. At certain points in life, we're all helpless in different ways but we recover, I said in my mind.

~6~

Gossiping

He did not come for work the coming week. Some of our coworkers were gossiping about him and his life. While some supported him others do not. Truly speaking, the ones who need to take up his work were not very happy. In that way, it seems they will spill any negative side of him should they know him more.

During lunchtime, I hang out alone. By the way, I never had lunch with him at one table. He chose to stay away from others. He often appeared reclusive, it was just because of work that he remains in contact with others.

It was just those few minutes I get to talk with him s we wait for lunchtime to get over. That too not every day mainly because I find the need to make friends or interact with other co-workers outside the workplace atmosphere so that I might get to know them more.

One day as we were seated in the nearby eatery joints, Tanu told me few things she knew about Jag. She did not prefer to talk about him. But as she often saw me talking with this guy, she simply ended up sharing few stories about him.

She overheard some of our senior co-workers stating that Jag was a divorcee, he has had some bad taste in women. He is not like that in the beginning. He hit out well with his co-workers at first. He even dated a woman from another workplace nearby. Yet he simply claimed it to be a rumor – he's not interested.

I would better understand him since he's losing his mind most of the time and having difficulty being committed to one person. He was pleasant to deal with. But then they saw a sudden change in this person.

At times he was very hard to deal with. His sincerity at work earned him good accolades among his colleagues. But soon they accused him of taking advantage of weaker women who are naive or simply swept off by his charm.

However, there is a contrast to this claim. Tanu claimed that Jag had once dated a woman who holds a high position in the office. She was witty and appeared to carry herself very well in society.

Still, some of them who knew about them can't believe what was happening. She has reached a marriageable age now. She gets irritated day by day. People believe Jag was simply juggling his luck until he falls out of luck. They even go on to say that he was simply living off of her and clinging to her so that he may have a future.

Since he never proposes to her they ended having a big fight which ended their fling. However, several of them who know both sides of the story claimed such things never happened. They were just friends. Or they may be more than friends.

'He hated women!' Tanu exclaimed. I asked her why did she bother about it. She told me that it bothered her to see women suffering. I am unsure why she gives me that statement.

'I don't think Jag intended to hurt anyone,' I keep going because I wanted to hear more from her. She is very strong in her opinion. According to her women should have the liberty to live on their own. They should not be, in any way, exploited by their male counterparts. There should be mutual co-existence between the genders. We need each other equally, she stated.

By now I can sense that our conversation is heading towards the topic of the gender equation. The new age women are very much aware of their rights. I appreciate that kind of approach.

However, all kinds of evil actions towards them are not the fault of the perpetrator.

In most cases, a male-dominated society is prevalent in several parts of the world. However, in the contemporary world, many activists are trying to change the perception of women in society.

They want higher payroll, a higher place in the social hierarchical system. They want equal respect in society. I heard that in some societies they should be made the heir of the family.

'We are into the basic issues of the society,' I said. 'Let's leave it at here today. When you discussed serious topics it is sometimes difficult to turn around into touches of humor in the end. Yet we're often able to do that. It is because someone has to agree with the other or at least show some decency.

~7~

'Where are you?'

Jag came back the following week. He looks refreshed. He is smiling at everyone when he enters our workplace. He put on his blue cardigan wrapping a small wool muffler around his neck. He seems to be in fine health. But when some of our co-workers casually asked him why he was not coming the previous week he revealed he visited a doctor.

I had my lunch and headed out to breathe in the outside air. The weather is changing fast. It was nearing winter by this time. Everyone was searching for sunlight. It seems strange how things have changed over a short period.

Then I saw Jag standing at the far end of the driveway. He was sliding his back on the concrete pole erected just for decoration. He did show any facial expression, not like the other days, when he saw me walking towards him. Today his blue cardigan shines bright in the sun.

He waved his hand at me signaling there is space beside him. I wanted to ask him what had happened to his health. But as usual, I waited for him to tell me. We talked about general things, which were happening around us.

Then he took out his phone to show me one social media post by a user. It reads: *'where are you? I hope you're somewhere alive and well.'* He did not want to show me the name of the user.

However, going by the glimpse I get as he swiped the screen, it goes something like *'thelostchild'* (the lost child). I ask him to show me once more but he politely refuses to do so.

By now I can almost read his mind. He is missing his child. Since his child as per my assumption can use social media accounts he or she must be in his or her late teens. 'I'm so sorry for her....' he said.

I got to know from him that he was following my short writings on that day. He told me how he wished to be that father who took his child to the village church rather than taking her anywhere else. There are many places a father can take his child. However, the first place he took his child would have a life-long influence on their children. I rebutted him for talking like a loser. 'You can still do it,' I said.

All of a sudden he burst out laughing. I am unsure whether these laughs truly come from the heart. I am perplexed by this sudden change of emotions. But it is Jag. So I need to bear with him. Many fathers had taken their children to the sanctuary of God to learn the ways of life. However, it is sad to see some children waylaid by the evil one who was lurking like a snake to swallow them.

He goes on to tell me that it was his child who wrote that post. Many times he wanted to reply or give a comment on her posts. But he dare not. He was not sure whether his only child would accept her as his father. He was afraid. He ran away from home leaving his young child and mother to live on their own. However, when he discovered that his child was on social media because his heart still beats for her, he decided to follow her using the name **'*bluecardigan*'** (blue cardigan).

He saw that she was searching for his father. She wants to see him very much. All her posts were pointing in one direction – the one who left her. Yet he wanted to act normal. His wife might be behind this. Sometimes the updates posted are too much to bear even for a grown man. She seems to be growing up in a huge vacuum.

'Just like you,' I remarked. But he acted as if I say nothing.

~8

No Comments

'**D**id you ever go back?' I asked. He did not give me a reply. I rephrased my question and asked him again and again. He simply smiled. Now I know I'm getting irritated too.

'Go away, that's how you wanted,' I continued. He turned towards the pole. 'Those were the words I last heard from home,' he said.

I reiterated that I am not interested in his story nor do I wanted to help him. I am busy with my own family. Sometimes, it's difficult to keep things fall in place. So I don't want to hear something which is not very inspiring. When I told him just like that, blatantly, he wanted to say something.

'Please Sam, don't do that. I will tell you one more thing. Hear me out. You might be the last person I'm telling all these things, said he begging. That was the first time, I saw him do it. Then he kept on narrating his story again.

He was not ready. I can see him simply stammering his words. It doesn't make sense talking to him now. I realized that it must a chapter in his life so far. Ostensibly, I try to keep away as far as possible. We talked about the people surrounding us in the workplace. He did not seem to enjoy the humor and presence of some co-workers although they claimed to be his friends. I made known to him it's better on my part not to comment about it. He is indeed very difficult to deal with at times, anyway.

As time went by I also interacted with many of my co-workers in the workplace. It's a beauty to meet tons of people with different mindsets and views. You cannot generalized people based on a certain story or things you read about their place of origin. A metropolitan city is rich in diversity. No one can claim it to be their own.

Some people gelled or adjusted too soon that they got lost somewhere in the middle. Yet some conservative people are rare yet firm on their values and belief. I enjoy people who know their roots and appreciate the roots of others.

I did not tell you this before: Jag is not religious. He is not an atheist. He is just somewhere there in the middle. I used to share my religious views and how I found peace and comfort in life. But it's the work of the spirit if he's to find the truth in life. My purpose is not to convince nor coerced anyone, not only him. His condition – living style and his peculiar connection with his family made him do that. Yes, he sometimes used 'peculiar' too many times in describing himself – his past and present.

Then what made him keep going? That's what I wanted to know as well. The look on his face when he shows me the picture of his child says a lot. I'm afraid that I might misinterpret his emotions. So, I hardly passed any comments whenever he talks about her.

Yet I have the assumption that he misses her very much. I don't know what he would like to do in the future or where did he see himself in the coming years.

Sometimes I want him to reconcile with his family who was physically and emotionally far far away from him. I don't want to go to that yet. All he knew about them was a broken-hearted picture of themselves in his mind.

In the time to come, and when he is ready, I hope he will put up his brave front towards mending the ties between them. From what I saw and heard so far he was fine with how things were going. But he also wanted to change his lifestyle – living alone in the city where there were lots of people around him yet he was still very much alone day in and day out.

~9~

Absentees

Every day is not a good day at work. One day a pile of files filled my desk because of the absence of many of our co-workers. The day seems long. Some of the work needs urgent attention. The scene was messy when you handle different works at a certain time.

There was hardly any help coming my way. All of us are busy with our assigned work. The files become an added pressure on us. This is frequent in a workplace that is poorly managed. I am waiting for our lunchtime to freshen up myself.

At last, it was lunchtime. I had my lunch on my seat quickly as I wanted to rush out so that I may get some fresh air. I was sitting there relentlessly when Jag also came out from the building and we sat again on the front patio of our office building.

He appeared cheerful today. I am not sure what had gotten onto him. By the way, he was unpredictable. It is possible that he is enjoying the pressure at work or he must be having a good dream the other night.

He came to lighten me up. He talked about various things ranging from his work experience to the unpleasant jokes he's heard so far. I was half-listening to him.

Today I need space. The sound of traffic behind us is deafening and disturbing to me. I have never really felt this way before.

Whenever he says something which is supposed to be a joke, I smiled. Their work experience sounds boring to me, there are too many changes between the past and the present scenario. I was like, please stop now, in my mind.

'Raise your children well, Sam,' he said to me all of a sudden.

This time he got my attention beyond the needed amount.

And soon I hit back:

'You are an absentee parent or father yourself, how can you lecture on me!' I almost raised my voice too loud.

His eyes almost popped out of his thick glass. Then his head and body stoop down towards the ground. I simply watch him. There is no feeling of remorse in me for a while. Then I saw certain people who overheard us staring at us.

They started to excuse themselves away from us. By now, I realized I was going too far. But the damage has already been done. I wanted to say sorry but I did not. He simply smiles trying to regain his composure.

After a period of silence or being absorbed in the deafening sound of the road traffic at its peak, we're back to talking terms again. I made a brief apology which is followed by him. He also admitted that I was right to a certain degree.

However, he reiterated that if I were him I'd do the same thing. We met a different person in life, some are committed while some are not. But then I make another stand: it is not always an issue of commitment but adjustments and fulfilling our obligations when it comes to two persons who try to live together.

Taking him as an absentee father and husband, I want to know what is his future expectations for his child. He never hardly give a good thought, was his reply. That kind of thinking simply hurt him in his everyday life.

He was just a ship sailing where the wind is blowing although there are times he seeks contentment. Contentment seems to be far away from him.

Tanu wasn't interested in this story. But I often share it with her. She is sure that she does not want such type of a person who does not care about his wife. According to her, the husband must fine-tune his marriage or his relationship with someone he was committed to.

I have to agree with her. By the way, I am just agreeing with both the sides and their viewpoint. A woman does need care and loves more than a man. Some women claimed to be stronger than their male counterparts. They have this mindset of being able to live by themselves.

Gender equation ruled on them and they fight for it. Here I am afraid to tell you about the subject as I will not be able to give justice on the subject.

However, Tanu is not the kind of person who is one-sided. She is determined but not extreme. Yet she did not like the story of Jag very well based on what we know until now. There must be more to it.

At the same time, she was afraid his story might influence me in the wrong way. We also wanted to know more if he would like to open more about himself.

To me, the story is an escapist from the hectic working atmosphere. Tanu knows how to extract a humorous way of telling stories. Her jokes are sometimes boring to me though.

Sometimes it's a pity how our co-workers would often make fun of Jag although not in a way disrespecting him. Valentine's day is a good occasion for it. We would hire an old lady for him to bring him rose on that day. He knows it is us who did it. However, he would painstakingly burst out into his laughter as if saying, 'no, not again!'

He must have hated the old lady but he seems delighted to see us happy more than him. It is a gentle reminder of the roses he had missed since he was away from home. In that way, Jag gelled well with different kinds of people around him. It seems all of us wanted him to return home because by now except for the new joinings we know a part of him.

Just to make him feel good I told him he is clear on what he is doing. And that's a good point to start with by not letting him affect that much. He was adamant to believe me at first.

So I go on to say that there were parents who live at home with their young ones but never paying attention to them. It's a living hell for their children.

They are setting the wrong example as the children are observing them closely at what they are doing. With no intention to build a home that will serve as a foundation for the next generation, they are breaking the home piece by piece.

Looking at me in great despair, he seems to be lost as to whether it makes him feel god or reminding his role as a husband and father. Living as a community is in our instinct. Far more than that caring for a small home that we acquired is more important. It remains true for men and women. Some of us keep breaking the ground but never built a sure foundation on it.

~10~

Closed chapter

Our Director called me one day. This time there is a need to meet our possible new client in another city. An extension of a business is on the way. She told me to go on a trip with Jag being my senior who first contacted them before I joined this workplace. However, Jag's changing attitude has to be covered in some way.

She told me that I might have the chance to take over Jag's role in the near future should our meeting goes well. I have a feeling that it was meant to be a motivation for me. But I do not want to overtake Jag in his current role. I would like to take over her place only. Just saying!

At first, I am reluctant to go on the said business trip. I have a young child at home. I will miss them. But since it's work-related I inform my wife. Then we decided I will go on the trip as per the requirements of my workplace. I don't know about Jag —how he feels.

He was there already checking our files. The will be a learning experience for me. When we reach our destination, we were busy with the scheduled meeting. Our meeting went well despite the unusual or queer humorous ways of describing things by Jag. It seems I might be the only one who finds it strange. The other party in our meeting seems to enjoy his way of conducting himself.

We were able to finish the meeting quite well. It will be on my records as well as his. But I'm not so sure about the credibility of the party we met. We have just one day before our scheduled return. Jag told me there was a closed chapter of his life he wanted to re-open. I'm not sure what to expect. But late into the night, he narrated from the first night he left home.

On that night when he turned his back towards his home because he does not want to disturb his wife and child sleeping peacefully. He went on looking at the wide sky he has no thoughts. His mind just went blank. As he walked into the streets a flash of light coming from what seems to be a vehicle keeps following him.

The source of light becomes nearer and until it comes to a halt near him. A fellow whom he knew from playing a board game, sometimes gambling late into the night, appeared from the vehicle. They were surprised to see each other unexpectedly. The man asked him to go with him. Since he was heading nowhere Jag soon gets in the vehicle.

As they were deep into conversation, the man revealed that he was going to the neighboring country for business purposes. He further asked him if he would like to accompany him. Jag then unhesitatingly agrees to go with him. It was supposed to be for a day or two.

After a short time, they changed their vehicle. This time into a half-loaded minitruck.

They traveled the whole night. For his friend, it was not his first time. He was enthusiastic about their trip. He does not reveal to him whom they were meeting. From what he told him all he knew was they were dropping and picking up few goods from the border.

The next day, early in the morning, they reached the border. His friend told him that they need to cross the border. He was reluctant to go at first. But when his friend hesitated he was willing to go too. However, when he began searching for his Identity Card, he found out that he had none of the ATM cards, ID Cards. He only left them at home.

But his friend was able to arrange for him his entrance to the other side of the border. The man has frequented the place thus he knew the trade of doing things. Soon, they crossover to the other side. There they went to drop off the goods they were carrying. Since they have some time to enjoy themselves, they hang out in the nearby suburb.

His newfound friend wants him to join his trade stating it was hugely profitable. They talk about money and how to acquire them big. He became interested in the trade. His actual dream was to make some money for his dream project. However, he doesn't want to leave home in its entirety. The misunderstandings at the home front will soon undergo a makeover, he hoped.

There was one thing he did not know. For his friend, it might be a big hurdle if they return the next day. He has no proof of his identity. His friend was not expecting this from him. It means a cut from his earning as he will need to bribe the officials again. There is far more to it than what he knows.

By this time his friend had already work-out his plan of getting back without him. He assured Jag to stay there for a day or two or until his next trip. He also lends him some money. So, there's no immediate problem right now.

He simply has to wait for few days before his friend gets his identity cards or everything he needs from his wife. Then he will come back to pick him up. In the meantime, Jag will get acquainted with few people who might become his business partner.

It's what he did at best – his escape from the real world. He would not like it if I told him straight in his face. Many times I wonder what's going on in his mind as a father and a husband.

If it's me I'd missed my family very much. But if I am in his world I might be worse than him. After all, I don't want to judge.

~11~

Staying Away

His friend went back the next day as per their agreement. Jag did not mind staying away from home for a day or two. Who knows things might get change for good when he gets home. It was a vacation from his daily routine. If his wife misses him a little more...he thought to himself.

His friend did not return in a day or two. He waited for a week. Still, now news from his friend. Jag was not petrified. But when it completed two weeks his money almost get used up. Now, he went to the people his friend had dealt with.

They told him that he was arrested on his way home. There is a report about him transporting banned objects and narcotic materials. Someone has reported about his traveled plan. He was jailed. He became a high-profile criminal.

Even if his friend returns, he might have suspected him of reporting him. But after a year he came to know that he was reported by the person whom he dealt with in the first place. In the black market, this is not new. It happens everywhere.

Jag soon ran out of time and money. He has no identity in a foreign land. His dignity and integrity were lost. He ended up in the street begging. He slept there in the open. His clothes lose their colors. By now no one would recognize him just by a glance. He still hopes a missing report might be filed by his family. And then one day they will find him.

When begging was not enough to give him food he started to act like a fool. He ate whatever he saw. As he told me about this chapter of his life, he said he enjoyed it. I think he was being sarcastic. When you have nothing to lose and no fear of death because of your situation you simply lived without thinking much, he told me.

He wants somebody to hold him at night as he counted the stars so that he might sleep soon. It was a different world out there he says. Some months had passed by when one night he was awakened by the sound of a gang fight. He was afraid they might mistake him for someone and shot at him. So, he pretended to be sleeping in his begging spot.

One party had mistaken him to be one of their men. So, they took him home. When they reached the place they found out it was the wrong person. One of the leaders shouted at his men for picking up the wrong person.

On that night they lose one of their mates. The police took him away. When one of them suggested that they hand him over to the police, Jag cried for help. An illegal immigrant has no future in jail. He will be imprisoned for life. There is no one to stand for him.

So, they decided to put him back on the spot they found him. If he didn't go away and not report what he had been through in three weeks, they take him in. He was left in hunger in the open for another three weeks. He wasn't sure if these people are a lifeline for him.

Three weeks have passed. But no one appeared even in the shadow. He waited for another week. He is facing the real hard time of his life. At last, they took him in.

They asked him what he can do. 'I write songs,' he told them. There was no role for a songwriter in their business. Laughter filled the room. So, he too joined in.

'Can you sing too?' 'Yes, I will.
'No, are you good at singing?' I will sing.

They found him useless. Their business is not near around entertainment. As he pleaded, they took him in to accompany one team. This team deal in black marketing of gun.

Slowly and slowly, he was introduced to the business of the Golden Triangle. This becomes his entry point. Trading in guns has been a dangerous area. He learns the art of making a deal here. Although he claimed it is a different kind of a deal which involves a great deal of study and technicality.

He told me that delivering the goods is the most dangerous part of the execution. No one value your life, they value the goods more than us, he said. I am not interested in this thing. So, I told him to fast-forward. Still, he wants to tell me so many experiences. Yet I declined.

From there he moves onto the opium trade. He lived in the cultivation area. He works in the field – harvested it. The flowers are lovely but what they cause mankind is destructive. Its addiction looks painful. Most farm owners have either one or two addicted in their households. They earned money but also loses valuable young lives.

He also told me that he tried his hands in different fields once he owns multiple identity cards. Gold mines in the Golden Triangle are interesting, he said. I almost asked him whether he has gold in his name. But looking at his present situation, he doesn't seem to possess one.

All the narcotic drugs, flesh trade, and all kinds of evil that are happening in this area are hard to believe. He saw their *modus operandi.* He also advises me to stay alert and protect each other from the evil world. He saw money, gold, luxury, and also who almost acquire one of those but perish on the way. My words cannot describe what I went through, he mumbled.

'Fine! Did you go back?' I asked.

He goes onto tell me that he become more lonely with time. Now that he has the required documents he decided to go back home. He doesn't know what is he anticipating. But he wants to see his family. Things might get change and they may take him in.

'But how do you think they will survive all these years?'

'All my savings are with them. She is very determined. She'll live. I'm afraid she'll be better off without me!'

Having said that he wanted to continue more. But this time it will be his homecoming. I am also eager to hear about his determined wife again. I have the assumption that they are on good terms in the present time also.

He is not done with what he encountered in the *Golden Triangle*. But I am less interested in such things as cruelty done on people. It is not cruelty at first but when people are blinded by want of money, they care for nothing.

Making money at the behest of someone is a norm there. It is more like the saying, 'Do as the Romans when you are in Rome'. We are born natural predators but just a little bit civilized than other species.

Only the two of us are sitting on the balcony late into the night. Still, he whispers, 'Sam I too have managed a bank account in our neighboring countries. He doesn't want to reveal much. I don't want to know much about it. It is his hard-earned money.

'Good for you!' I commented.

To ease his pain while recalling his past I added that some men and women lived an equally different virtue at work and home.

Many diligent workers may not turn out to be good partners at home. But we can find at least one good quality in a person who did not live up to the obligations of the home and society. His wife too must have a very good side of her which I intended to hear about if given the chance.

~**12**~

Homecoming

Although he was unsure what awaited him in his home. He decided to quench his longtime pain of missing home. However, he was unwilling to gather information before he went home. Till this time it was not a planned life but he still survived through thick and thin.

Whatever lies ahead he will face it. He possesses the confidence and guts to face anything. Living alone for his life would do no good. Yet he was in a dilemma about what to expect on the back of his head. With all the documents he owned he applied for a visiting visa, which guarantee his entry. Once he reached home, there is a hope of reinstating his true identity.

He set out towards his home.

After a good day of traveling, he reached his old town. It changes a lot. Some of the streets saw a facelift. However, they're not beyond recognizable. Jag set his foot again there on the street where he was once picked up by his friend. A plethora of emotions filled him.

As he made his way towards his home, a neighbor saw him. He stared at him for quite a long time before he approached him. Jag was ashamed of his frame right now. His appearance in the territory where he once painted his face on the street becomes shameful.

He simply stood there for a while. His destination was just a few blocks away. The neighbor came to him. He wanted to confirm whether it was him, the old Jag who lives next door. He seemed very much surprised at first. But recompose himself.

'I will take you home,' he said.

They went towards his home knocked on the door of his house. The knocking sound felt like it sounded deep in his heart, almost unbearable to bear. He was lost about what to expect. His wife opened the door.

'Here, Jag has come back,' said my neighbor as he pushed me forward to enter my house.

'Jag who?'

'Your husband, let him in. Then we'll talk.'

So he entered his home after a long time. His wife kept on repeating that his husband was dead. Or at least to her, it seems. His neighbor quickly picked up the situation. He excused himself away. But to call him if the need arises.

A little girl from the corner observed all along. She was frightened at first. But soon realized he was his daddy. She came near him. Yet she was cautioned or signaled not to do so. There was complete silence in the house.

She was unable to hold her tears. They embrace each other. Their little girl joined them. Tears flowing all around. His wife must have so many things to say. She kept on saying why I did this to her. It would have been better if he did not return, she'd whisper as she kept away her tears.

However, it was worth the comeback. His sweet little child misses him a lot. Her laughter was infectious. It filled the room. Thus they all burst out into laughter. I believe it must be more like one of his vague smiles he often in the workplace and the laughter outside.

They settle down for the day. Each on their space - distance was maintained. They did not react nor started a conversation. There will be insurmountable questions.

In the wake of dawn, he inspected his old home. Everything was very much intact. There seems to be no outsider living in their home while he was away. His toolbox however seemed to be used occasionally as they did not rust that much for three to four years. Some of them need polishing.

He then emphasized the lives purely on mutual trust and respect. They have not revisited his past. It might blast out again sometime.

Jag never went out nor away from home. He wanted to rebuild his home. However, his home is doing well without him. His long absence made him alien to the new development. The lifestyle is hard to adapt to. But he is trying.

Time has passed by when he decided to run his bank statement. He wanted to know how his previous savings had been used during his absence. Previously, just before his disappearance, he was a dealer in a real estate agency. He remembered the savings he kept for his daughter's future and their next possible family business.

One day he went to the bank to run the statement. He came back discovering what he had expected. His wife is living off of his savings, hardly adding to it. It's a possibility that she holds another account. There are lots of transactions towards his in-laws. They had earned their degrees and are running their own business or non-governmental organizations. He was okay with it as they thought he was dead.

Jag then wanted to talk about it to his wife. He wanted to know if they need more money. At first, it was very difficult but if there is a need he wanted to transfer his foreign holdings on their savings. His wife took it otherwise. She wanted to hide how she used the money left behind by him.

'So what? We thought you're not returning. You're not there.' He understood the situation. He was unhappy nor happy with the way his earning has been spent. But they can leave it behind to start a new life.

However, the accusations of him having another family while he came up to the fore. He offered his explanation to all the queries his wife posed at him. It was a good development for them, unlike their first stint. Before his disappearance the problem is that they did not talk – all the charms in their love-life are fading.

He further told her his disappearance was not preplanned. It just happened. He was apologizing yet remorseful. Now his wife was missing his presence but not fully ready to accept him because of the pain he has caused. Her pain surpassed her melancholy once he reappeared on the scene. And they already found a way of living without him.

By that time, words had soon reached his in-laws. They are not ready to admit their utilization of Jag's savings. Repayment was not on their mind. They blamed him for leaving their young sister. He was kept almost like a house-arrest in his house.

His in-laws guarded him well. They don't want him to go any further. His wife was given the pressure to contain him. For him, it was a time well spent with his child. He was afraid his longing for the outside world might overtake his thoughts again.

He soon became restless. They saw his weak point – if they could turn him to the police with his foreign documents and deny hide his identity card he could stay another good time in the prison. This time, his wife was not ready to do it. But the pressure is mounting on her. So, she hid the identity of him which he did not explore until now as they live on mutual trust.

They turn him over to the police! I was shocked when he revealed this incident to me. However, he shed no tears. I saw no change in his emotions. He wants to keep going on narrating what has happened next. But I wasn't!

How can this happen to him over and over again? It is one of the many hardships he faces on this earth – both at home and in a foreign land. He simply told me that it was better here in our home country. I have to agree with it although I have no experience in this matter.

Soon it became the reunion of him and his friend. His friend who was on trial for a long time now was jailed there too. He heard about him through the lawyer of his old friend as Jag was locked up in the same place.

His old friend has a long record of illegal trading and activity along the borderline. He was operative around the Golden Triangle and even boasts of having connections in the Golden Crescent to other parts of the world. He was in the position of hiring good lawyers but it was difficult to get him out.

Throughout their short meeting, just before he was transferred to a larger facility, he remained apologetic. But they did even utter a single word about where they met and their modus operandi. If officials overhear them taking of such things, it will further worsen the case for Jag as well.

His old friend promised him that his lawyer will soon bail him out. It will be his way of him saying sorry for what had happened due to their traveling together on that fateful night. Jag told him he will forever remain grateful if he keeps his words. Soon his old friend was transferred to another larger facility to serve a longer period of his term.

~13~

Trust Deficit

After being away for such a long time with no traces of him, the trust deficit is normal although they were now under the same roof. He tries to put things back on track. It's not as easy as it looks. The most important element in marriage – trust - here between them is missing. This is mostly the missing link of a relationship that went through turmoil.

I learn this from people I have met before. The movies, books, and almost everything is talking about this deficit.

He went back to state one fault line of theirs when they started. That is – not to believe what anyone says about them, they were trying to make a circle of trust without addressing the missing link. If they heard what people were gossiping about their past, it would be better they have to address it first hand. And that too till they fully regain trust.

Without this trust in a relationship, there will always be trouble. Uncleared past issues are often the biggest hurdle to a relationship. To gain full trust, they must clear all their doubts and not be afraid of losing each other.

Jag further told me that he was not comfortable, in other words, afraid that they might not be able to accept each other anymore.

In all those years while they were not together, he cannot depend on the reports from their neighbors. There might be more to it or lesser to it.

She was not sure whether he comes clean. Why didn't he bother to establish contact while he was away? His answer to this was already presented as per him. He was living on odd jobs without a proper identity.

Truly speaking, he's hiding as he was hiding because he did not want to serve jail term in another country. He might get stuck there forever. There must be other reasons for it too.

Once he got to establish an identity he came back, that's according to him. He thinks he does not owe an explanation more than that – it was those dark years of his that he does not want to visit often. He even referred to it as the 'Closed Chapter'.

'You could've open that closed chapter to your wife fully so that he might believe you.' I said.

'There were things beyond what she would believe in me.'

'Now that's your problem. And that is one reason why there is a trust deficit under your roof,' I added again.

He told me that he was not bothering her with what had happened and what is not happening nor was he judging on the way she spent his savings thinking that he was not returning anymore.

'Are you speaking the truth?' No

I assumed you don't want to know everything. He does not agree with me on this. He was afraid that his only chance to live together again might go down the drain again.

He was afraid. Truly speaking, he could not afford to go alone again – but in the future, if he goes alone again, he will be very determined – one night he made up his mind although he did think of disappearing once again. The first was not preplanned – it should not occur again...

Then it might be worse than the first.

At a certain period, she wanted him to undergo several tests if he is free from any kind of transmissible disease. This hits him hard in his heart. He would never do it, he was clean according to him. He stays as a married man even though he was away.

This will be their first step of sharing the bed again. He got furious – he asked the same thing needs to be done with her. She was not reluctant. 'I will do it. Let's get tested,' she was confident.

However, he does not tell me whether they did it or not.

I told him that I was not interested in their bedroom stories.

Yet he continued, 'I got tested,' he said. 'and all's well.' He continued.

Again I told him to keep it at that. At the same time, I think it's good he cleared all the doubts about this one in the least.

I am expecting good progress in their story. But he did not go on to tell me anything. One thing or another came up in their story.

'No, we have our good times as well.' He said. Yet his emotions tell the opposite.

~14~

If you are a man

His neighbor knows them well. He kept taunting them, 'If you're a man maintain peace inside your home. It's a challenge that was intended to serve good for them.

They began to hate their neighbor. Their neighbor was getting fed up with their behavior. It's not his business but he was very much concerned about their future. From the time, Jag returns home he was expecting a new development in them.

However, they are not reading him very well. His intention towards them they did not know. They thought that he was after their property. They mistook his intention to be as if they get a divorce he will be acquiring their property.

As a neighbor, he was very much concerned about the example they were setting in the neighborhood. He never was eyeing for their property.

Once he got to asked Jag about his time in the Golden Triangle, he was reluctant to reveal it to him.

'If you need money earn for yourself!' he said to him without much thinking. His neighbor has no intention to go there. He was a different person from him as he never gambles. He was trying to raise a good family.

However, he was intrigued by how Jag had spent his time there for so long. Jag did not want to go into details either.

He told him that he worked very hard while he was there so that when he could return he would be able to open his own business with a huge sum of money.

People he met there were either very poor or very rich. Most of the businesses were run by certain tycoons who rose from nothing while some inherited from their parents. One thing he did found out to be strange was that most of them got stuck once they enter the business area.

Most of the newcomers were treated very badly. However, those who are coming by their choice were either in a do-or-die situation.

Many of the underdogs make it big there yet with a big price to pay. Especially those who wanted to leave early like he had to lose huge amounts of their earnings once they decided to leave.

'You will not want to be there,' he concluded after narrating a part of his story to him.

His neighbor again made a challenge: 'You have survived there. I am very happy for you. You are a man. Now if you are a man, it's time you maintain your small well. Seek peace in your home. You cannot stay forever this way.'

He agreed. Yet as usual he did not appreciate such kind of advice from a person whom he found to be self-righteous.

To end their conversation, he simply told him that he was working very hard on it. But inside him, he was taking the challenge or advice in the wrong way.

I don't know what happened to this person – how he looks cool today and his unrelenting past – presents a big contrast of personality on this person.

I almost wanted to ask him how he's brought up. But other times he told me that he grew up in a good family. If so, then he must be the black sheep. I keep it to myself. One has to know how to divert the topic of our conversation anytime when you're with this kind of person.

One more thing I saw in him was that he was very bold in his perception and presenting his ideas – in work-related matters and outside. He hates politics very much that even when we talk about it he was almost cursing as he read the newspaper.

That's strange to me.

His reaction to certain topics or the way he reacted to certain advice makes me think that he might be emotionally volatile due to some reasons which were unknown to me.

I would very much recommend he meet a therapist. But he would never agree to it. So it was better said than done, in his case.

His story till now makes me think that there might be a solution to this person's problem. If I could help him well in the future, although I'm not a learned person in this matter, I could see him regain his life with his family.

~15~

The Blue Cardigan

Jag was out again. He went home again as he felt he cannot stay away for the rest of his life. However, external influences caused turbulence in the sailing of their journey. He wants to makes the most useful time of it. He wanted to make memories.

Keeping aside everything at bay, he devoted his time to building his home again. Yet certain things came up again. It was difficult for his wife to neglect his past. His wife wanted someone by his side while he was away. So she trained their child in a way that even if he returns, she will side her mother in everything.

Thus their daughter loses respect for her father. He became a nuisance to their existence. One fault of his wife, as I observed, is that in her wishes to build her home or finding support, she is breaking their home. Their child is lost between them. She did not know which way is right. The atmosphere at home changes dramatically, which made him think that his absence might be better.

'So you run away again,' I interrupted.

'I beg to differ. It's an adjustment.' He replied.

Then we debated that he was only trying to justify himself. We talk for a longer period this time again. He wanted to tell me one more thing. His empty laughter ensued. When he regained his composure, he reiterated that his 'Blue Cardigan' is a reminder of the new development.

When he told his wife about his willingness to leave home. She seems okay with it. Yet she remained sarcastic in all her comments. I was surprised! To me, was so wrong to think about it again after they lost some good time a few years ago. It becomes their way of life.

'Anita bought me the Blue Cardigan,' he said as he took a deep breath as if submersing his life story so far. He was not sure whether it was meant to be a parting gift or a gift for his lost valentine.

He never mentioned her name until now. Something unexplainable must be going on deep in his mind. He seems very much disturbed but when I confronted him, he simply told me that he will keep his integrity intact instead.

He wore the blue cardigan while walking his daughter in the morning as evening. His daughter clings to him. The innocent daughter of his would never understand what was going on between her dear parents. She would one day understand when all will be revealed in her mind.

'It's your ego otherwise,' I hit back. He remained silent. He was adamant to talk. I give him time. It must be a clash of ego or just the unforgiving hearts, which gets hardened in due course of time. He keeps focusing on himself saying it's his personal life. So I may not comment on it. He was in pain.

He looked far towards the empty sky:

O birds of the sky,
Flying high in the sky
Together you fly high
Have you ever been
Ever been weighed down
Weigh down by
your heavy heart?

Fly high O birds
Never look down
Take me with you
Make me feel lighter
O birds of the sky
Fly, fly, fly, fly.....

He sang something like this. Flying high on each of their own does not seem to give him happiness. Each he talked about his journey, he kept singing a song that goes on this line.

Their upbringing called them to be different. 'Adjustments' seems to be the other word for defeat. None of them can withstand correction. Both are determined in their ways. Their conversation about almost everything ended on a sour note. It's never like before they get married.

If that is the case, he thought they should straighten their career path. None of them wanted to sacrifice their egoistic nature. Also, Jag can stay home and surrender his dreams. But he cannot afford to do that. Anita is also focused on her dream to remain independent. They both have worked very hard to get to this level.

Family for them is not necessarily living together. The practice of 'Single Mothers' and 'Single Fathers' in society is doing the rounds if they could afford to raise their child by themselves.

I saw this personal trait in him too. And as per his story and description, his wife seems to possess the same personal trait. So when they are together there is an equal action and reaction.

Love is tough for them. Adjustments can go both ways, humbling or disappearing from the scene.

We can choose any one of them. To ease his pain, I told him that I almost chose his way too.

As I try to leave him there on the balcony, he called me back.

'Please contact my daughter for me. Follow her on social media and befriend her. I missed her so much.'

Going by the social media post he has last shown to me, she seems to be missing her father too. So I agree with his request. And if it turns out well, it will be the beginning of their reconciliation. He even told me that there's no one more than me who knows about him and his family. It will take time to fulfill his request. But it might be worth a try.

We take our trip back to our workplace. In the next few days, a new working strategy and partnership were put on the table. In the meantime, I told my wife what I have heard about the story and the strange request. She supported me.

So I started following the **thelostchild** on social media. I am waiting for the right time to DM her. It will take time for her to get acquainted with me. I don't want to rush. If she was like me she might not trust anyone on social media. But every time she posted about her father I try to draw her attention.

In the meantime, Jag was required to live in another city where we met our new client to oversee our full connection with them.

Our Director asked me to filled-in his place. I was unaware of this new development coming up when our Director told me that I will take Jag's place. She further went onto say I might get her spot one day. She is joking about the remark I had passed when she told me to join Jag on our first trip to the other city.

Coming back to *thelostchild,* Jag was encouraging me to go faster in contacting her. I came to know that she might want to meet her father. There is a huge void left by her father. She also believes that her father would somehow read her posts because some of them were meant to be addressed to him.

One day I dropped her a private message saying, 'I know where your father is and who he is.' She did not reply. The message was already delivered and shown as read. I don't know if it was actually her who read it.

Jag kept asking me whether I could establish contacts with her. I did the same to him as his daughter is doing. I did not reply.

'Kindly send a picture of my dad if you really know him,' popped a message on my device one day. I was almost reluctant but since Jag had asked me I cannot keep it to myself or simply betray him. So I sent her a picture of me and her daddy on our last business trip. I captioned: a strange yet very warm person.

She hardly replies to me. I don't want to rush her. But I often dropped her a message stating that I could arrange their meeting in case they're willing to do so. And also told her to keep it private for now. She has to act cautiously. I told her that too. If her mother was against it. It will be aborted.

~16~

The Lost Child

Sonam agrees to meet her father someday. I'm sorry I did not reveal her name earlier than this. It's because I was not sure if that's her real name. His father Jag uses a different name for her. And now I realized it's his way of calling their children in adoration.

She did not tell me when will that happen. I told her, 'the earlier the better.' With that note, I also sent her a picture of my visiting card. I inform the new development to Jag as well. His voice defines his excitement in meeting her. However, at the end of each call, he was somehow afraid that she may not fully accept him as her true father. I waited for her call.

It's a matter of time for their meeting. I passed on every information, other than Jag's location, to both of them. No one can rush on other's life when you find it difficult to it on yourself. But for this father-daughter duo, I wished they'd meet soon. In that way, it would be the starting point for their reconciliation or worse the end of it.

We're not in the same workplace anymore, a city apart. Sometimes I thought it's better to end our ties. But seeing what he has gone through in their life, they deserve to meet again even if it is for the last time.

One day a call came to our workplace. Someone is asking for me – a lady. Tanu picked the common line. She transferred the line to me. She looked at me as if I'd done something wrong.

'Not your wife!' I can read her lips. She gave me this deadly look on.

When I answer the phone I wasn't surprised why she did that. It's Sonam who is calling.

'Call me on my number....' I give her my contact number. Right now I'm occupied with my work. I don't know what to expect when she calls again. After that, I explained the new development to Tanu.

It's not what she was thinking. I did not learn the art of making *close friends* outside my marriage. She is protective because she is afraid Jag might be an influence in a way she did not want. I appreciate it. But she can mind her business. It was fun though.

Another week has gone by. No calls of any sort have come yet. I am expecting it. I wanted to put this story out of my hand. I thought that if I could establish contact with one of his family members, they might be willing to accept him. Yet sometimes I doubt it.

I am also afraid about the kind of people I'm going to meet. If the father has this character, I don't know what to expect. But I have to finish it. I have to heal them if I could.

I am waiting for the call again. What if her mother is not permitting her to do it anymore. For the sake of their father who is not yet dying I hope they'll meet again one day, even without my presence.

At last, I received the call. She wanted to talk to me in person. But she did not know to specify when and how....'Why are these people so unpredictable?! She simply hangs up the call, giving me no chance to speak.

~**17**~

From home

Since she knows the city I lived in, she called me all of a sudden.

'I'm coming tomorrow.'

'With whom, how...?'

There's no reply. It's difficult to inform my family. We need to get ready. What kind of person is coming tomorrow. If any untoward incident arises how am I going to handle the situation. I called Jag to tell him her daughter is coming. He too did not say much. Yet he seems happy as there's a chance to meet her in the coming days.

Jag asked me about her itinerary. I did not know either. He was more nervous if she happens to come with her mother.

'I don't care. It's your family. You must help me if I face any difficulty in handling her.' I told him. He assured me that he would. Looking at his past and personal life, it's difficult to trust but his way of dedication in the workplace makes me believe it.

The next morning, before I am going to work, Sonam called me. She has arrived. She will be staying the day with one of her friends and I do not need to worry for her. It gives me a huge sigh of relief. I don't like when people say anything to keep to myself.

'Do not tell anything to my father yet. I want to talk with you.'

'Sure, we will meet in the evening.'

I called Jag about the new development. Since the weekend is approaching he must be ready to meet us when I call him. I also instructed him to come back and stay in the same city as us for a few days. His previous PG Hostel might take him in.

Sonam and I met in the evening. I invited her to our place. It's her first time in the metropolis, she was polished. She looks smart. Just going by her first impression, she would do well if she searches for a job here in New Delhi. Although one problem here is that few people are lucky to earn in good numbers.

And as we talk slowly as we sip a glass of tea, she started asking questions about his father. She has very few memories of him yet talked very fondly of him. I don't know where to start. I am waiting for her to reveal more.

She was hard-headed. This time she wouldn't go back without meeting her father. The void he left behind in their home was beyond repair. People bully her, tease her as the one who did not have a father. If it was not for his neighbor who once took Jag into the house, life would be very difficult for her. He treated her like her own daughter as he has a daughter almost the same age as her.

Their neighbor's daughter was her best friend in their schooling days and beyond. She can recall crying late into the night thinking her father would meet come and protect her. But to her disappointment, her father did return once but to leave her again which leaves a scar deep in her heart. She longed for fatherly love.

As we listen to her story, sometimes she can't control herself. I was afraid she might become violent because her soft speaking nature dramatically changes as she was deep into her memories. I wanted to pat her on her back but I acted cautiously so that my touch of comfort might not be mistaken.

She was apologetic in nature because of her childhood trauma. We feel for her, we must handle her carefully. I asked her if meeting her father would help him. She was unsure. While at home, she wasn't allowed to talk much about his father. She kept it at her heart only. So we revisited more of her memories so that she may get healed up to some extent.

She was into her late teenage years. She was mocked that no man would like her to be their wife. She and her mother were left by her father as they were unable to cooperate with her father. Who would like this kind of woman to be their in-laws.

At some level, I saw there's a sense of relief in her eyes. When the authority in the house did not work together you cannot expect their ward to be disciplined very well although it depends on the person. It's in the heart of a man or woman to determine their character.

We decided that she will meet her father the next day. There is no change in her facial expression. She's been there facing all the hard times in her life. She has only one hope – meeting her father might ease things up.

~18~

Preparing

As we're about to take rest for the night, she told me one thing that she believed was done by her father. Every month or two since she had her bank account, some amount gets deposited on her account.

'Oh, that was me!' I joked. She would not believe it. There's a suspect, and we hope it's true. We'll get to know you soon. I am not sure if she can sleep that night. She was dialing her mother's when I get up to sleep.

They would talk for very long hours. Her mother must have become more protective. She'd be afraid of losing her as well. The day before she set out for her long-standing journey, she was told to return home. She'd let go of her if the situation demands – that's what she told me. I hardly believe it.

There's a reason for her mother to do it. And I agree with her. I would say her mother must have been really determined. What Jag had told me about her before, now I am getting some glimpse of it. As for me, my wish is for them to get back together at any cost.

The next morning I called Jag so that I might be able to set them up. He told them that would be possible in the evening. I was somehow afraid he might run away again. However, in the back of my mind, I think that he was willing to meet her only one beloved daughter. There are several things he wants to clear before they meet.

I asked Sonam several things to clear up. She told me that Anita. Her mother and herself lived in the house now. Most of their maternal uncle had grown up. They did not visit them again as often as before. They earned their living, they were married off, having their family to look after.

It was not as her mother had planned before. Once their uncles get married off her mother get to know she was on the wrong side of her life. She would never admit it either.

Somehow I have this feeling that she might want to get back to start a new life with Jag. Taking things into consideration their breach of trust would be very difficult to mend. It is as if their glass heart had cracked. Not only crack but has fallen into pieces.

In the meantime, I also believe that if Jag has no will for things to fall back into place again, he might never revisit his dark days with me. Yet I also saw that he became lighter when he sees me.

At first, I told you that he is not religious. When I met with his daughter, she told me that he was a very good young gentleman who was pipped to serve God in the future. 'He is promising,' people around the neighborhood would tell Sonam. She simply whispered, 'I wished,' in her mind.

Some of them blame her mother for destroying him. While her mother's side was strongly against this notion of gossiping doing the rounds. I asked her what she thinks of it. She did not want to comment on that. 'You have to meet my mother,' then you'll know because by then you'll be the best person to know about them.

She did not want to believe that his father's time in the Golden Triangle was not preplanned. Her mother could not believe it either. Yet her mother was always unwilling to give the reason why her father did it. I wanted to know whether she would be able to forgive her father.

'I wanted to meet him first!'

'Fair enough,' I replied. She wasn't naive. I could not read her mind. I could not imagine myself in her shoes. Both the parents – her foundations are undecided - meaning not stable. But as I saw her, her determination and lessons she learned from the life she might not be willing to go through would have given her some wisdom of life.

Their journey was more complex than I first think about it. I also reveal something about her father to her, which I hope would help her as I am preparing the ground for a father-daughter reunion. By this time, if she was revealing her true perception of the matter to me, she might be ready to meet him.

'If anything happens when you meet your father, please do not pass any bad comment on him. Anyway, he is your father. You should respect your father. I am not on anyone's side. I only wanted you to make peace in this short life.'

She agreed with me. But she seems to be a little bit frightened when I said this to her. I have to assure her it is not for her to fear anything. Somehow I was afraid to take all responsibility on this matter. I have this feeling their reunion would be the beginning of their family coming together again after so many years.

Sonam asked me if she could meet her friend during the daytime. There are some places she wanted to visit in the city. Although I do not know who her friends were, I agree with her. She has to meet me again in the afternoon before the sun went down. I am also nervous about this meeting.

~19~

It's about time

It's about time they have to meet now. I am waiting for Jag to call me when he was ready. Since it's their affair I wanted him to set up the place and everything needed for it. He told me he would do it as expected of a man.

His call never came. The evening was approaching, I don't want them to miss this rare opportunity of meeting each other. I assured Jag that his daughter was respecting him or at least wanted to see his current status.

Sonam called me up telling me she was about to meet me. I told her to come although I have this strange feeling their meet might not happen as planned. I called for the second time, he did not answer the calls. He might be running away. Most of the time he was uncomfortable talking about his family.

His daughter almost arrives at the place where we were supposed to meet. It's a small restaurant set up near a huge park. I intended that if they're uncomfortable to meet or talk in a place filled with people although they might not be interested in their family story, they'd move to a park. There, they can have an isolated conversation by themselves.

It makes me frustrated when he did pay attention to my calls. It was just for him, if he wasn't ready why did he started this in the first place. I began to doubt his existence- the existence of such a person. I was thinking it might just be a facade I was talking to all this time.

But he was real since he eats and dines with me during our trips. However, his unpredictability makes me doubt this person from time to time.

It was because of this strange behavior of him I started talking to him in the first place. He was different. Yet this is not the time for him to act this way. His daughter whom he wanted to meet will be meeting him.

He has to regain his composure – his staying away might be hitting hard on him right now. Sometimes blood relations are the most difficult ones to meet due to the mixed emotions one has had.

Truly speaking, I cannot say much about how their meeting would turn out to be. It might be the start of a new chapter in their life or the end of their long-anticipated dream meeting.

I could somehow measure the emotions flying between them. Yet he has to answer my call or it's about time he calls me now.

Nevertheless, I am positive I will be able to arrange their meeting. Sonam was on her way to meet me. She was almost here. I don't want to brief

her anymore. Let them meet in their true sense –
no formalities, I said to myself.

Somehow, I wanted to witness their meeting too.
So, I set out with Sonam to our destination where
Jag sent me the address. It was a holiday in the
middle of weekdays. There's not much traffic today.
We reached the place. We waited. Sonam started to
feel something is wrong. She was apologetic and at
the same time doubting me whether I was just a
person who played on her emotion.

Many times I had to assure her that Jag himself
had requested me to do this. Once she began to
doubt me, I really hate that feeling. She must be
insecure right now – she's alone here with me.
What if I am doing was one of those that Jag had
seen during his time in *the Golden Triangle* and *the
Golden Crescent*.

No, I will never do that to this young and gentle
woman who's already lost in this big world. She has
parents who did not pay attention to her. I don't
want her to curse her birth anymore.

All that bullies she'd been through was too much
already. It's about time her life must be put back on
the right course or what was supposed to be.

However, she was sitting waiting with me. It's
about the time his father came into the picture. So,
I called her father again.

This time he answered my call in a hush-hush
voice. He told me he has to rush back to his
workplace the same evening as there is an
emergency coming up in the other city where he

works. I was left astonished! I don't know what to tell her daughter. Worst, she might be afraid of me now!

She looked at me blankly. I could not look back! Now, it's about time I have to do something.

~**20**~

On the Driveway

Just then an idea struck my mind. I can enquire about him to his old PG owner where Jag used to stay while he was in New Delhi. She might know his whereabouts or I hope he must be putting up there whenever he visited our city.

He is very well attached to this city since it's the place he can find solitary life without any disturbances. Mostly in the evening, he's likely to stroll or sit in the corner of a big park.

I called the PG hostel owner who confirms Jag is there. So, I told Sonam to get in the cab, to meet his long-lost father. And we hurried away into the deafening sound of the traffic. By now she is somehow uncomfortable – she looked nervous. Anyway, she's lost in whether to trust me or she will be meeting her father.

'We would soon reach him,' I said breaking the silence. She gave me a smile from her rather sad or weary-eyed face. She must have trusted me.

When we reached Jag's PG hostel, he was there standing on the driveway with his traveling bag. I assumed he was about the leave the place. We were just on time. If not, he might have left the city going back to the other city where he was working.

'Why did you do this to me?' I argued when we pulled up in front of him. I don't know if he was doing this to me or his daughter. Sonam stands beside me holds the corner of my shirt. Jag seemed surprised to meet me there.

'Here meet your daughter!'

Jag recomposed himself, he tries to wear a smile on his face. Sonam understood the situation. She went forward and tightly hugged his father. Tears ensued.

I give them their space as I excuse myself to talk with the owner of the PG hostel. The hostel owner did not know what was going on. I did not bother to tell her either. Yet she was very much curious to know.

If she'd be of help in the future, I'll spill some of the beans to her too. But not now. I simply told her they were meeting after a long time. It's the first for her to know he has a family somewhere.

'I've been willing to meet you all my life,' said Jag's daughter. He has nothing to say to her. No excuse this time around. He looked at her all grown up – his daughter who had grown up in his absence the absentee father he was.

'I am very sorry. I know sorry isn't enough right now.' He replied.

'But dad, if you may let me call you, why are you still running?'

I don't want to interrupt them. I am also wondering where he is headed. Had we not come in time, we would have missed him. We intercepted him on the driveway. 'Why is he so fond of the driveway?' I said to myself as it's the first place in front of our workplace where I met him for the first time.

Then I suggested we have a cup of coffee together somewhere. They agreed. I ushered them inside my vehicle. As we drive out, I told Jag that I will drop him off after a while if he is going to another city. He told me that he wasn't.

'I wish this will be the first time you met and not the last time.' I told them. This time Sonam's face lightens up a bit. She might begin to trust me. And I told her that her father was also very trustworthy in the workplace. He is a good person.

Yet Jag was still apologetic stating that if he was a good person all this would not have happened.

'How's your mother? I asked Sonam. Silence entered the scene. I understood the situation. 'Oh, maybe later, not now!' I continued.

I wanted them to bond over a cup of coffee – their first after so many years. Sonam reiterated how much they missed a father figure in the house. Jag looked uncomfortable. I tried to excuse myself. But he requested because I knew it already.

'There's a very long story about your father,' I started. It will take a long time to fully recover from the past. I wanted Sonam to say something good.

His father was acting in his best form. I want them to grab the situation for their best future.

'Many people talked about how good my father is, she said. 'I still believed he was such a good person. So I wanted to meet him in person.'

Her father began admitting his mistakes and how things get out of control. He even considered ending up unknown to anyone forever. However, he saw himself in another light. He did not want to destroy himself. So he started working as he wanted to support his young daughter. It's his way of admitting that he was the one who sent money to her now and then.

'Whatever it is you will always be my father!' This statement brought tears to Jag. He appeared older than when I first met him. He kept repeating that he was very sorry. He could not give her the best gift as a responsible father would.

But his daughter assured him that she has no bitter feeling towards him. There must be something she did not know that was going on while she was a child. This time I saw the character of a grownup in her.

'Father, do not feel bad. Let's forget our past. I will try to talk to my mother for our reunion.'

The night was growing old. So I decided to leave them. But Sonam reckons she will be going back with me. When I glanced at Jag for his opinion, he seemed okay. I told Jag to stay put in the city so that they will get to meet more often before she turns back to her mother.

As we headed home again Sonam expressed her happiness in bringing back his father to her life. Although they may not live together, she now knows she can meet his father more often. Her happiness knew no bounds. She was ecstatic and excited to tell the new development to my family.

'I am going to give you a new task,'

'What would that be? She looked surprised.

'It's your turn to bring your father home or prepare your mother so that they'd meet again before it's too late.'

Then I also told her how I worked or get acquainted with his father to reach this point in his life. Family is the most important unit of society. If it breaks we cannot simply look at them without doing something. The next morning she was ready to return to the Geyzing suburb area in the Himalayan region.

She thanked me over and over again while I keep reminding her of her next move. I also reiterated that in any case, she fails to convince any of them, it should not affect her life. The show must go on.

The running father was met on the driveway, I whispered to myself. By this time, I believe there would be certain progress on their reunion. However, I try my best to distance myself from their family affair as I also think that it's about time they had to reroute their journey.

~21~

Relieved

No one bothers to contact me again. I feel very much relieved. Let me reiterate here again that I have no intention of interfering in someone's life. But I saw this as an opportunity I cannot deny to help someone in need. I hear him out all through his pains.

He would still have lots of things to tell me. His posting in another city in one way is a relief for me.

During our lunchtime, I got to hear how our coworkers knew about his story. Most of them were half-truth if the narration of his story to me were to be taken as the truth. As far as I am concerned I believed his story. Had we worked on his family in the very beginning, his life could have been very different. He was and still is very promising to this day.

I recalled our meeting with his daughter – how hard yet easy when we were together. It's his character that sets him apart from others. He is in some way not interested in mending his old ways. Yet he is not ready to assassinate himself for that matter.

I wanted to meet his wife but I was afraid he might seek help from me again.

In the fast pace of life, we did not have time for others. I have to focus on my career as well. I wanted to rise the hierarchical ladder in my workplace too. For that, I need support from my family.

One day Jag called me. He told me how relieved he was to meet his daughter. That 'hug' from his daughter gives him the will to live more. He goes on to tell me that he will be calling his daughter often.

'It's time you meet her mother too,' I added. He did not respond. I continued, 'alright, work on it.' Now that he has a new sense of living, he was relieved and very delighted to meet me again once he visited the city where I now resided.

Life's a journey, I might move onto different places if the situation demands. However, there is a longing for a place where I can call home – my birthplace in the countryside.

Sonam called me up from time to time. I do not ask about her mother. She also told me that she's very much relieved now that his father established contact with her. One sad thing she told me was that her father is still reluctant to meet them at home.

'Why not your mother come here with you once?' I enquired. She was hesitant to reply. Later she told me that that's what she was working on right now. In the meantime, she wanted to enjoy the new freedom of her heart – at least her father is in a distance where she can call him when she wanted to.

Moreover, I advised her to stay strong and not committed the same mistake – I called it a mistake because she put it that way. Her father did not want to relate to it as a mistake rather it's a choice or adjustments to survived both of them and their marriage.

Jag never asked me for my opinion. So he took it as I agree with him in his choice of life. If he's a writer, I think he would write the best lyrics out of his life. Most of the beautiful and touching lyrics of a song stemmed out from the heart of a sufferer or melancholic person. In his part. It will be his pain, which leads him to his first odd jobs and establishing his life again in the city.

~**22**~

Seeking Peace

All of us were busy like others who were working to put bread on the table for their family. One night he called me. It was time for me to take a rest. I rebuked him. There'll be nothing very important nor a hurried matter with him. He talks slow and he acts slowly while it comes to his personal life.

'Please call me at the appropriate time,' I told him, by that I mean it's better to call during the day. When someone is at home it's mostly family time. He should understand that. Everybody is not like him. Although I reminded him many times regarding the best time for his call, somehow I felt guilty today.

'Anything you wanted to say, please?' I asked him.

'I wanted to make peace with my past!' he quipped.

It's very difficult to comprehend him. I'm not sure whether he meant it or not. Moreover, if he stays true to his word what would be his likely next step. Does he mean to seek peace with his family? That must be one of them. If so, will he go back to meet them again? I'm not so sure.

'Did you ever asked about Anita to your daughter?' I asked again. He told me that it'll be better to meet me in person. So I told him he can meet me over a cup of coffee when he is ready. He is in his thinking mood. You never know whether he really meant it or not. Also being his call coming in late at night. He must be sitting alone somewhere on the terrace of a building reflecting at his past. If he comes I would meet him.

The next day he called to inform me that he had booked a reservation at Barista Expresso Bar in Friends Colony. We agreed to meet there after work. Since it is far from my workplace I was hesitant a first. However, the meeting might be meaningful to both of us as he was seeking peace which could end up as our last meeting, I am positive of the outcome.

He expressed his willingness to make peace with his past. I had observed a few changes in his appearance and trait – his age or some other thing must be catching upon him. He informed me that his daughter kept in touch with him.

She also visited him in his workplace. I wanted to ask about what his wife's reaction would be. But I waited as he narrated their contacts and the development in their way of the reunion so far. Forgetting each other is far from reality although they might not be together.

He was unwilling but his daughter wanted them to be patched up. Anita was not very responsive. Every time they try to establish a conversation she was busy with her work due to the heavy influx of tourists around March, April, May, and June.

However, Sonam told him that her mother was ready. Jag wanted her to come and visit him first. Yet she was hesitant. She would be home instead of that. On the back of his head, Jag told me that he had this fear of rejection or avoidance once he reaches home.

Further, if they were to live a separate life there, it would be better for him to stay away. He found things complicated. He cannot be away throughout his lifetime at least for Sonam as she nagged him by and by.

Then I encouraged him to go forward and work his way out of his workplace. I also suggested it will be good for him to go at the onset of winter. As we're living here in a very hot summer season, it would be wise to set out before winter arrived there in their hometown according to him. I have never been there so whatever he thinks would be best for him.

Leaving that aside, I am very excited about his willingness to seek peace after this long year of living a solitary life. If his life gets healed again he would be very privileged as a father, husband, and for himself.

'I forgot to bring something for you,' he said

'Never mind, when we meet again you can bring it for me,' I replied without thinking much. He was a delight to meet with always. His way of laughing at small jokes of mine and his best compliment of me saying, 'you're always smiling, Sam' although I might not be brings joy to me. At least I appeared that way to him.

As we sipped the last cup of our coffee, we noticed time has skipped past us today. It's time to go home for us. He would go to his old Paying Guest Hostel and I will go home. We bid goodbye.

'Thank you for everything!' he patted my back while his cab arrived.

'You don't need to....'I shouted back as his cab whizzed past me.

My greatest wish for him is that he finds peace in his life again as was expected by us. And that will be the end of his old story – for a new chapter will begin.

~23~

Something for you

Since they did not bother me anymore I thought they might be enjoying their reunion now. They deserved it. A happy family reunion awaited them per my perception.

'I have something for you,' Sonam told me on the phone. 'I wanted to meet you again.'

'Let me know when you are coming.' I did not inquire much about the reason why she called me after almost seven months. I assume that their dysfunctional family has been patched up.

Till today, no one spread the news of Jag retiring from work. We heard the news from one or the other, sometimes the unlikely hearing about our co-workers who retired or worked in another city. So I took it as 'no news means good news.

Jag's daughter never showed her emotions in her voice. She had dealt with it already according to her. She is strong and at times unpredictable. She loses control over herself but she tends to hide everything in her. She's still very self-conscious – at times insecure, if I could help her I want her to over all of these. Yet I know her for too little nor do I saw her normal self in their hometown ever.

Whenever she calls me, it always left me wondering where she and her family are headed. But as I laid out before, I wanted to finished what I have come to be a part of their journey in a good way.

'It's an envelope from my mother,.....or us,' she told me.

'You can open it and sent a picture of it,' I replied. 'You can send to me by post as well,' I continued. She did not give me a quick reply. It seems she was whispering to someone else. When you are on a call, it's somehow uncomfortable if the user on the other end did this to you.

'I will come to deliver it by myself.' She told me at last. It was in the year 2019 now. I assumed it must be something very important or that matters to them.

~**24**~

Final Homecoming

Spring season has arrived. The eye is pleased to see the new life springing up from those left behind by the harsh winter. It is considered one of the best times here in New Delhi.

There were, and there will be flowers blooming in the gardens, on the roadside, and the *Gol Chakkar(s)* or the roundabouts in several parts of the city.

Sonam too arrived in the city. She will go back the next day to help her in their family business. I love her hardworking spirit. In that way, she seems to take much from her father.

I want to know what is that thing she brought from me. She took out herbs and indigenous spices from her bag, which her mother packed for us.

Then she took out an envelope from her bag and give it to me. As I open the envelope, there were two things inside: One is a banker's check with a very big amount endorsed to my name. I was thrilled. Second, there is an envelope which I am very familiar with bearing the logo of my workplace.

My familiarity with the envelope prompts me to open it sooner than I ought to. There is a handwritten letter inside it. It reads:

Dear Friend and Good Listener,

When you read this letter I will be finally home. I wanted you to have this letter as your token of my gratitude to you. Although I can call or meet you in person, I want you to have it this way. (my apologies)

I wanted to thank you for everything you did for me. Meeting you during lunchtime was an opportunity to heal me as you help me revisit my past to seek peace with the people who are dear to me.

I would like to start over if given the chance had we met earlier. I am hoping my wife and my only daughter would appreciate your work as well.

(I looked at her daughter happily as I read this.)

Here is fifty percent of my possession which I saved during my time away from home.
Please accept the amount, but the date and encashed it for you and your family so that you will be able to spend more time with your family. The amount will be enough for you to start something in your name. I am not trying to repay

your time with money but it's a token of my gratitude.

Sincerely,

Jag - The man with a story
September 5, 2018

'Well, I am very happy for you. But I will not be accepting this check. I will endorse it your name.' I told Sonam.

The look on her face this time is very strange to me. There's something not known to me yet. When she is ready she will tell me. I don't want to rush someone before they're ready. And the same thing goes for me.

'You will have to accept this so that my father would rest peacefully.' She told me. As I waited she slowly told me that his father was homed finally. I told her that I wanted to know more.

On September 8, 2018, Jag set out for his home. He did inform them that he was going home to meet them. And that they will live together forever. The next day, was an incessant rainfall in the area that led to their home.

The Highway was affected by a massive landslide, which is common in the area. The vehicle which Jag has boarded got stuck in between the landslides. They were not washed away luckily. However, they could not move forward nor go back to the nearby village.

He was determined to get home after a long time. This becomes a new obstacle. He was near to his hometown but unable to move forward.

When the rain gets thinner, they walk on foot to crossover the muddy terrain carrying their goods by themselves. By now Jag is past his prime. And as they trekked the slope of the mountain, he accidentally slipped away. He slipped down till the base of the mountain.

They searched for him till darkness sets in. They were unable to locate him yet. Words reached their home soon. His wife and daughter were hopeful he could be rescued.

Late into the night, they found him. With the help of the villager nearby they brought him home.

His Blue Cardigan was turned into muddy brown color. Poor Jag's plan did not go well. He went into a coma. He did not speak. His fever is running high for three consecutive days.

Sonam shed her tears as she narrated what has happened to them. I was left speechless!

On the third night, his condition was getting better. They all slept peacefully. There was peace in their home after a long time. They have a father and a husband.

But in the morning Jag did not respond to anything!

They opened his traveling bag, there was a gift for both of them. At the bottom of his bag was a photo of them pasted together sharing a hearty laugh on the day he was gifted the Blue Cardigan.

He's home forever!

సౌసౌసౌ

~**25**~

Epilogue

In the brevity of life, all of us are writing our stories. Many of our stories have touched lives in different ways. Some people start well and finished well.

❧ ❧ ❧

About the Author

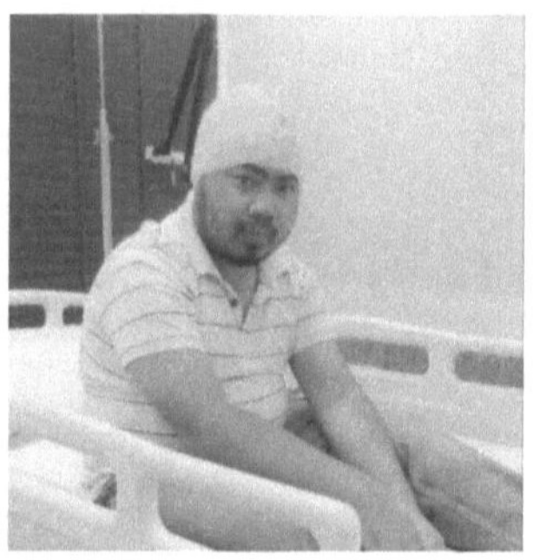

S.Thuam Siam Ngaihte @ Siam Ngaihte is a writer, Indie author, and blogger on life memories and inspired topics. He is now fighting a certain *neurological disorder* for more than a decade. He is a former banker at State Bank of India, a husband, and a father at home. Brought up in the countryside of Northeastern India, his family now lives in New Delhi, India.

Other Works by the Same Author

1. Unconsumed: In His Abiding Grace
2. Walking Outside the Garden
3. From the Sideline (Upcoming)

www.abidings.com

ॐॐॐ